INNER-CITY DIET

Maurice Patterson

Brooklyn, NY

ISBN: 978-0-557-72219-8

Author: Maurice Patterson
Editor: K. J. Reilly

Acknowledgements

"To everyone looking to improve their health."

Contents

INTRODUCTION

Inner-City Diet takes a candid look at the perilous eating habits prevalent in the low-income, urban communities, and walks the reader through the process of exchanging their unhealthy choices for those that are healthy. The author breaks down the calorie count, fat and sugar content found in the typical inner-city meals and explains the negative impact it will have on your health. The workbook style questionnaire, suggested exercises and diet plan is an excellent way to get motivated to take the first steps toward a healthier lifestyle.

1

THE QUESTION

THE QUESTION

Let's get right to the point. I invite you over for dinner and when it is time to eat, I serve you the food I cooked but I eat something else. What would you think? You would think there is something wrong with the food I'm serving you and you would be right. Now, go to any Chinese restaurant in your neighborhood and look at the food they're eating. Have you ever seen them eat four chicken wings and fried rice? Have you ever seen any of the workers or owners of a Chinese restaurant eat barbeque spare rib tips? Have you ever seen them eat General Tso's Chicken? Whatever that is, because who is General Tso and why do you want to eat his chicken anyway? The key point here is that the families that work in Chinese restaurants located in the inner-city don't eat what they serve us. Could it be because they are aware of the long-term side effects of eating this type of food, which include high cholesterol, high blood pressure, obesity and a whole host of other ailments?

The Chinese restaurants and other fast food restaurants are selling us death tickets and they don't care. They gain financially, while we gain weight and develop health problems. These types of restaurants and other fast food establishments have scoped out an excellent source of revenue preying on the ignorance of the poor. Many of us are too happy to fork over our cash to make them prosperous, and make ourselves sick. The intention of this book is to bring awareness to the serious issues surrounding the deteriorating health of minorities, due to poor nutrition and lack of exercise. I aim to help the urban consumer from poor communities change their eating habits. We will start by taking a look at the various food establishments in our neighborhoods.

ASK YOURSELF

Have you ever asked yourself, why so many of us living in urban areas overweight? Why do we suffer from diabetes, high blood pressure and high cholesterol? Is it in what we are eating or drinking? Well, if you choose both you are correct. In the inner-cities, we eat and drink the wrong things. Most of the food we consume are high in calories, highly processed, full of sugar and deep fried in oil. This includes both the food we eat at fast food restaurants and food we indulge in at home. A lot of the so-called soul food we eat is destroying our health, making us obese and clogging up our arteries. We are, in essence, setting our souls up on the express line back to our maker.

I'm not saying that you have to stop eating the food you love, but cut down on the size of the portions. Instead of eating the entire carton of french fries, eat half. By cutting your portions you will lose weight, even without exercising. Weight loss has more to do with how much you eat, not how often you work out. If you work out every day but still eat the same amount of food you were eating before, you will lose weight very gradually. This is not necessarily a bad thing. However, in order for us to reverse our ailments, we have to be vigilant about what (and how much) we are putting into our bodies, particularly because it is the root cause of our health problems. Once we are able to identify our eating fallacies, we should correct them and we will soon reap the benefits of good health.

MY STORY

Between 1998 and 2001, I went from 180lbs to 270lbs. I could not believe my weight gain and did not know where it came from. Later on I found out that it was because of my poor eating habits, which I refer to as the inner-city diet. As far as I was concerned, I did not eat much - at least that is what I thought. At the time, I ate three meals a day, which we all grew up believing we were supposed to do. So, since I was not eating five times a day, or pigging out at the all-you-can-eat buffets, I thought I was on point. But apparently, I was not. Here's a glimpse of what I was actually eating everyday:

Meal	Description
Breakfast	McDonald's Breakfast
Lunch	A slice of pizza and a soda
Dinner	Chinese food (*Broccoli, white rice and garlic sauce*) and a soda

On the surface, the meals don't seem like such a huge amount of calories, but when you add them up it's another story altogether. The average human is supposed to get 2,000 to 2,500 calories a day. However, if your goal is to lose weight, then your intake should be approximately 1200 to 1800 calories each day. When I added up *my* average daily food intake, it was close to 4,000 calories. To gain a pound of weight you have to eat 3500 calories, so I was pretty much gaining a pound and a half every week for three years. Having said that, let's take a closer look at the food I ate with the calories posted.

Meal	Description	Calories
Breakfast	McDonald's Breakfast	1,150
Lunch	A slice of pizza and a soda	290 and 250 calories respectively
Dinner	Chinese food: Broccoli in garlic sauce, white rice & Soda	2000 and 250 calories respectively

MY PICTURES

It took me less than 3 years to go from 180 lbs to 270 lbs.

Before: at 180 lbs   Later: at 270 lbs

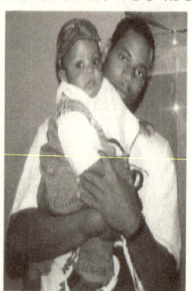
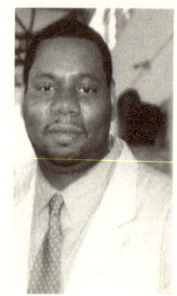

THEN AND NOW

Since then, I began re-educating myself about what I should be putting into my body. As a result of getting a firm grip on the value of healthy eating and exercise, and putting it into practice, I am down to 220 lbs and looking to lose 20 more pounds. After figuring out the cause of my weight gain, I adjusted my eating habits. I realized that my weight gain was due to eating too much fast food, french fries, white bread and white rice, so I cut my portions. Also, I had to cut down on soda and soft drinks, which are major causes of weight gain. The high content of sugar in soda not only impacts weight gain, but increases the risk of becoming diabetic. In the past, I would drink two sodas a day, but now I drink one soda or soft drink a week. I replaced the soda and soft drinks with water, which has zero calories. Additionally, I removed all of the large plates from my house and kept the small ones, so that I could cut my food portions. You may not have to go that far, but that is what helped me during the adjustment period.

Below, is a list of things that I do every day to help me in my on-going quest to lose weight.

- Work out 2-3 times a week
- Get colonic irrigations (quarterly)
- Count calories (See pages 37-38 for Calorie Chart)
- Do not eat after 9 pm
- Eat small portions of fast food (not more than once a week)

Fast food, french fries, white bread and white rice cause excessive weight gain. You do not have to remove them completely from your diet, just cut the frequency and the portions you consume. So, instead of eating a plate of white rice, eat a cup of white rice, or switch to brown or wild rice. Instead of having two slices of white bread, have 1 slice of bread, or consider switching to whole grain bread. Follow the above advice and your weight will drop dramatically.

What we put into our bodies determine if we are going to live a long healthy life or a short sickly one. What we need is re-education or what I call "health-ucation," which will help us take the first steps to making vast improvements in our overall health, and reverse our negative diets.

SIDE EFFECTS OF EATING THE WRONG FOODS

- Obesity
- High blood pressure
- High cholesterol
- Heart Disease
- Stoke
- Diabetes
- Osteoarthritis

WHAT CAUSES THE ABOVE AILMENTS?

1. Poor eating habits
2. Over eating
3. Eating before you go to bed
4. Fried Food (French fries, fried chicken, fried fish, fried rice)
5. Junk Food (Potato chips, candy, cookies, etc.)
6. Soda and soft drinks
7. Excess amounts of salt, sugar and calories
8. Lack of exercise
9. Lack of water consumption

2

WHAT ARE YOU EATING?

WHAT ARE YOU EATING?

A study conducted by the Associated Press states that Chinese restaurant food is unhealthy and loaded with salt, fat and empty calories. This includes the vegetables.

See article at: http://www.nbcnews.com/id/17718517/ns/health-diet_and_nutrition/t/chinese-restaurant-food-unhealthy-study-says/

The majority of food served in Chinese restaurants are deep fried, saturated with oil and jam-packed with salt. Chinese restaurant food is not good for you. Most of the so-called healthy dishes contain just as much calories as the regular meals. Plus, since Chinese restaurants are owned individually they do not have to post their food calories, or concern themselves with the same regulatory restrictions as chain restaurants or franchises.

In addition to the high calorie food served at Chinese restaurants, they offer the extremely high calorie sauces. Sauces like the Sweet BBQ sauce that we like to add on top of our chicken wings and french fries. This sauce is 30 calories a teaspoon and they drench our food with it, which adds an additional 200 – 300 calories to our meals. The hot sauce we put on our Chinese food, that's already high in sodium, is 130 mg of salt a teaspoon. So, this adds an additional 600 – 700 mg of salt to our meals.

For Example: Adding Sweet BBQ and hot sauce to your order of 4 chicken wings and French fries adds an additional 400 calories and 360 mg of salt to your dish. Now, instead of eating a 1700 calorie dish with 2200 mg of sodium, you are eating a 2200 calorie dish with 2560 mg of sodium. In order to maintain a healthy weight, the average adult should eat 2000 calories and 40 mg of sodium per day. Therefore, when looking at the calorie intake for this one meal, we are well over our daily quota. Particularly, when you consider that there are two other meals to be accounted for.

Additionally, the sauce, the vegetables and meat are cooked and saturated with oil and salt, which is very unhealthy.

My intention in this chapter is not to single out the Chinese restaurants, but to expose all of the deadly restaurants in the inner-city. Besides the Chinese restaurant, I have to include all fried chicken and burger fast food establishments, pizza parlors and the corner stores or bodegas. The inner-city diet, which includes Chinese food, fast food, Oodles of Noodles and other junk food, have an overabundance of refined white sugar, salt and oil. These factors are the number one causes of diabetes, high blood pressure and high cholesterol in poor communities throughout this country. There are many other elements in overly processed, fast food such as additives, preservatives, dyes and chemicals that help to speed up the process of destroying our health. Therefore, most of the places we purchase food from are co-conspirators in this path of destruction, but we have to take most of the blame for not guarding our most precious commodity.... our health.

CORNER STORE OR BODEGA

Go into any corner store or bodega in the inner-city and you will find it jam packed with nothing but junk food. As soon as you enter the front door you are bombarded with candy, cookies and cakes, which are nicely displayed in the store, along with the cat lounging on the bread. If you had no intentions of purchasing junk food, too bad, because that is all they're selling. Also, they have a small display of healthy food like the rotten apples, oranges and bananas. Oh, I forgot to mention the dried up lemons.

When you order a sandwich, you have a choice of an oil filled egg sandwich or mayonnaise drenched hero. Also displayed, are the refrigerators offering a large selection of sodas and soft drinks. Since there are not a lot of healthy selections, choose wisely.

PIZZA PARLOR

Are two slices of pizza and a soda a real deal? Maybe, financially but when it comes to your health it's a raw deal. One slice of pizza from the pizzeria is approximately 370 calories and that depends on how much oil, cheese and dough the pizzeria uses. So, two slices of pizza is 740 calories and add an additional 250 calories for the soda; that's a whopping 990 calories. Instead of calling it the pizza parlor they should rename it the funeral parlor because that is exactly where you are headed if you keep eating like that.

Other favorites available at the pizzeria are garlic knots and the old greasy beef patty with cheese. These foods do not add anything to our health, so if you must have them indulge moderately. Instead of eating two slices of pizza, eat one and give one away. Have a bottle of water instead of a soda. If you follow the above eating method you would cut your calorie intake by 620 calories. This will help you lose weight and look good.

LOCAL FRIED CHICKEN ESTABLISHMENTS

The local fried chicken establishments serve up a host of deep fried, oil filled and high calorie dishes, which consist of the following:

- Chicken wings (Fried in old grease)
- French Fries (Fried in old grease)
- Onion Rings (Fried in old grease)
- Mozzarella Sticks (Fried in old grease)
- Cheese Burgers (Fried on an old dirty grill)
- Sweet Potato Pie
- Ice Cream
- Milk Shake

None of the above foods are healthy and that's a shame.

LOCAL PANCAKE HOUSE

On Sundays, a lot of us take a trip to our local pancake house for a special treat. The food at this establishment is filled with so many calories that the establishment will not post the true calories on the menus. They only provide a calorie estimate. This is a clever scheme they cooked up to avoid scaring away customers with the real information, while still being relatively compliant with the Food and Drug Administration. This is outrageous! If you ever took your car to an auto mechanic, you know how estimates go. All I have to say about the calories at your local pancake establishment is listed below. Read it and weep. Remember the calories are an estimate, so there are more calories in each dish than posted.

- Garden Omelet (**1150 cal.**) What kind of vegetables are they using?
- Stuffed French Toast Combo (**1476 cal.**) This will help you combine those two stomachs you will have after consuming this meal too frequently.
- Harvest Grain and Nut Healthy Combo (**560 cal.**) The calories are low but check out the sodium (1090 mg). How healthy is that?
- Kids Funny Face Pancakes (**1456 cal.**) Now, who's laughing?
- Banana Nut Pancakes with Banana Syrup (**957 cal.**) That's bananas.
- Country-fried Steak and Eggs (**1480 - 1660 cal.**) PLEASE STOP!

The list of high calorie foods are endless.

BBQ FAST FOOD ESTABLISHMENTS

BBQ fast food establishments are another place we frequently go to after church on Sunday and on special occasions, like birthdays and holidays. We treat ourselves to some deserving food which caters to our unique taste buds. Although the food taste good it is very unhealthy.

> **Note:** I called a BBQ establishment located in Chelsea, NY on June 8, 2009 at 11:01 am and was told that they do not post their true calories on the menu. What do they have to hide?

BBQ, where the B.B.Q stands for "**Big Belly Quick.**"

JUNK FOOD

A lot of food mentioned in this book can be considered junk food, but junk food has fewer calories than most of the food mentioned. A bag of potato chips (150 cal.), a chocolate candy bar (250 cal.), and a slice of cake (305 cal.) has less calories than a BBQ Bacon Cheeseburger with Fries (1510 cal.) from your local BBQ or pancake house. In no way am I suggesting that you switch your diet to junk food, but I would like to bring awareness that candy, cookies and chips are not the only types of food that are considered junk food.

Would you get up in the morning and grab a bag of chips (150 cal.), a soda (250 cal.) and a candy bar (250 cal.) and eat it for Breakfast? No. So, why do you get up in the morning and go to a fast food burger establishment and order a breakfast that's 1100 cal.? What's the difference? The junk foods we purchase from the corner store are no different from the junk foods we order from fast food restaurants. All of it has negative effects on our health, and ultimately our life span.

SUPERMARKET

My mother had 10 children and we grew up on welfare. So, naturally, my mother had to purchase cheaper brands of food when shopping at the supermarket. Cheap foods have more calories, salt, additives and sugar added to them than noticeable items. If you do not believe me, go to your neighborhood supermarket and compare the labels of the cheap food to the brand names and gourmet items. To your amazement, you will find that cheap food has more calories, fat and salt and other additives than higher quality and gourmet foods. This is also true for condiments like salt. Cheap salt has more sodium than name brand salt, or the unprocessed sea salt, which is much more expensive.

I grew up on Oodles of Noodles (chicken favor), which are high in calories (380 cal.) and super high in salt (790 mg.). Unfortunately, sometimes we had to make do with what we had. We can make our noodles healthier by using fewer noodles and seasoning and adding veggies. Also, we can buy regular string spaghetti noodles and make them ourselves from scratch. For instance, you can cook the noodles in low sodium chicken or vegetable broth, and add steamed veggies and enjoy a healthy, inexpensive, low sodium meal, without preservatives or additives. Granted, it may seem drastic to go from instant (just add water) products to cooking your meals from scratch, but it's not as difficult as it seems. Nevertheless, it is important to point out to you that there is always a healthier option.

SOUL FOOD

Soul food, this is a very touchy subject. I grew up on soul food, I love soul food and I still eat soul food. I use to eat it in large quantities, but now I eat it in moderation. I eat smaller portions and add fruits and vegetables, which make the dishes healthier.

Most soul food dishes are deep fried in oil, consist of sugar, too much salt and are high in carbs and calories. This includes all of the favorites like:

> **Fried Chicken, Macaroni and Cheese, Potato Salad, Corn Bread, Sweet Potato Pie, Candy Yams with marshmallow, Peach Cobbler, Biscuits, etc.**

The statement, "You are what you eat," is totally true. Whatever you put in your body ultimately affects you in a negative or positive way. The foods that we ingest are affecting us in such a negative way. It is shortening our life span and causing us numerous medical problems. If eaten in moderation, soul food or any food is not a major health risk. The health problems arise when you overindulge on a consistent basis – week after week, year after year.

CEREAL/POP TARTS/CINNABON

Most people in the inner-city start their day off with what we are taught is a "balanced breakfast" that consists of a bowl of cereal and milk. This would be a healthy idea if the cereal we consumed was not filled with so much sugar, artificial flavors and preservatives. Below is a list of cereals that line the supermarkets we frequent and the amount of sugar included.

Brand Name	Amount	Sugar
Frosted Flakes	1 cup	15 grams
Captain Crunch	1 cup	18 grams
Fruity Pebbles	1 cup	15 grams
Apple Jacks	1 cup	15 grams
Fruit Loops	1 cup	13 grams
Lucky Charms	1 cup	14 grams
Pop Tarts (Frosted Strawberry/2)	2 pop tarts	36 grams
Cinnabon Cinnamon Roll (813 calories)	1	55 grams

The American Health Association recommends that women consume no more than 25 grams of sugar per day and men consume no more than

38 grams of sugar per day. While the World Health Organization recommends no more than 25 grams per day. If you consume a bowl of the above cereals, two Pop Tarts, or one Cinnabon, you have reached your maximum recommended daily allowance. Sugar is one of the number one causes of obesity and diabetes.

The number of children suffering with obesity has risen to over 50% in the past 15 years. This is the result of the processed foods, fast food, excessive amount of soda and candy and not getting enough exercise. Accordingly, 30% of children between the ages of 10 and 17 are overweight or obese (source: Business Week, 2009). The same article stated that on average, 25% of adults are overweight or obese. This number increases dramatically when looking at minorities in urban communities nationwide.

WHITE BREAD & WHITE RICE

Too much white bread and white rice are responsible for a lot of the ailments that afflict us. The negative effects of these foods include:

- Excessive production of sugar which causes diabetes
- Weight gain which causes stroke and heart attacks
- Heart disease
- Depression

White bread and white rice are highly processed foods that are depleted of any nutrients, vitamins or minerals. They are refined carbohydrates that your body turns into sugar. Instead of eating white bread and white rice, eat whole wheat or multi-grain breads and brown or wild rice.

EAT THIS	GET THAT
Too much red meat	Foul body odor, heart disease, increased risk of colon cancer
Too much fried food ,margarine & butter	Stroke, heart attack, high cholesterol
Too much sugar	Diabetes, depression, mood swings
Too much salt	High blood pressure & headaches
Too much white bread and rice	Weight gain and diabetes
Too much junk food	Cavities and weight gain, bad skin
Too much soda and candy	Weight gain, diabetes & cavities, bad skin
Too much potato chips & chocolate	Heart Burn, high blood pressure
Too much milk	Excessive mucus build up in the sinuses and elsewhere in the body
Too much macaroni, pasta & bread	Constipation, diabetes
Too much alcohol	Bad breath, liver disease, kidney and irreversible brain damage

3

WHAT ARE YOU DRINKING?

WHAT ARE YOU DRINKING?

Sodas, soft drinks and fruit drinks are filled with lots of empty calories, and additives that promote weight gain. They are primarily loaded with sugar, corn syrup, dyes, preservatives and additives. Most of the so-called fruit drinks have less than 10% juice and that's from concentrate. That means that most soft drinks are made of a very small proportion of juice and the remaining 90% of the soft drink is water, sugar, dyes, chemicals and preservatives.

The best thing to drink is water. We have all heard the saying "water is good for you". Why? Because our bodies are made up of 60% water, our brains are made up of 90% water. That's why our bodies require pure water to function properly. We need water to replenish and hydrate our system. In the inner-cities, we say we don't drink water because it's nasty, or it doesn't have any flavor. This is because we have grown accustomed to sugary drinks. In order for us to make adjustment to drinking water again, we have to, gradually, replace one of our sugary drinks with a bottle of water. Over time you will come to appreciate the thirst quenching, pure characteristics of water, especially when you begin exercising. Nothing satisfies your thirst better than water after a rigorous workout.

QUARTER WATER

When I was a kid, quarter water was the drink of choice because it only cost a quarter. It was cheap and it quenched your thirst after a long day of running around and playing in the streets (I wish more children did that today). This drink, that most children in the neighborhood preferred, was nothing but water mixed with food coloring and sugar. It does not have any nutritional value.

FIFTY CENT SODAS

If you're from the inner-city you know about sodas that cost fifty cents. They come in a variety of flavors: orange, grape, cola, ginger ale, etc. These sodas are cheap and very bad for your health. They are filled with sugar, food coloring and preservatives. A 20 ounce fifty cent grape soda has 30 grams of sugar and is 300 calories. That's 60 extra calories compared to the brand name sodas.

The combination of sugar and calories included in these sodas are making us fat and causing us numerous health problems. One of the major health problems facing minorities is diabetes, which is running rampant in urban communities. So, if you think you are getting a great bargain by paying 50 cents for one of these harmful drinks, you are not.

FRUIT JUICES

A lot of the so-called fruit juices we purchase for our children at the corner store or supermarket are not healthy. Most of them have more sugar and calories than soda. Below is a list of these so-called healthy fruit juices:

- Juicy-Juice(Slim Size) – 93 calories/22 grams of natural sugar (100% Juice)
- Capri Sun(cup)-120 calories/20 grams of processed sugar (no artificial ingredients)
- Ocean Spray(cup) – 140 calories/34 grams of sugar (processed and natural sugars, it varies from product-to-product)

After viewing the above so-called healthy juices you should want to stop giving them to your children on a regular basis. These juices should be given in moderation.

Make sure you are checking the labels on all products. Hi-C (for example) is not a juice. It is basically sugar water with dyes, and vitamin C. So quite naturally, you should NOT be giving this product to your child because it can be damaging to their developing immune system. Too much sugar for children can also groom them for craving higher levels of sugar as adults.

SODA

Soda is definitely not good for you. It's filled with acid, sugar and artificial flavors. Diabetes is one of the many diseases that will develop when you consume too much sugar on a regular basis, which will eventually take its toll on your liver. The domino effect on your health is nothing short of a horror story.

When I was young, my Grandmother used grape soda to clean her oven. It left the oven sparkling clean. If she could clean a dirty, greasy oven with soda, imagine what it is doing to your insides.

Soda Label Truth

- 20 oz. soda
- The nutrition facts state that the serving size is 100 calories.
- 8 oz of the soda is 100 calories, so we don't realize that there are $2^1/_2$ servings in this 20 oz bottle: 8+8+4=20. This means 20 oz of soda is actually 250 calories.
- Besides the calories, the soda has 69 grams of sugar, which is extremely high. The recommended amount of sugar per day is 25 grams for women and 38 grams for men.

Nutrition Facts

Serving
Size 8 fl oz

Amount Per
Serving
Calories 100

Sugar 69 grams

BEER/ LIQUOR

What do you find on every other corner in inner-city or urban communities? You find a Chinese restaurant or a liquor store. Some Chinese restaurants in the inner-city sell liquor. So, along with the calorie laced dishes, you can get a pint of cirrhosis of the liver.

Liquor and beer causes the stomach to swell and it damages your internal organs, specifically your liver. The liver eliminates harmful chemicals from the body. Without it, your body is prone to all types of diseases.

Liver dysfunction is often the result of alcoholism, and/or a side effect of diabetes. This is a serious concern. Without a properly functioning liver, one has to have dialysis every week, sometimes twice a week. Dialysis is a blood transfusion that is needed since the liver is not filtering the blood of toxins and pollutants. Otherwise, in a matter of weeks, your body would be

plagued with infections and toxins that will eventually lead to your system

shutting down completely. After spending less than six months without a

functioning liver, or dialysis, you will deteriorate to a virtual vegetable, until

you take your last breath shortly thereafter.   Trust me, it is not pretty.

4

CALORIES IN FOOD

CALORIE IN FOOD

CANDY BARS	CALORIES	DRINKS	CALORIES
Baby Ruth	280	Soda (20 oz Bottle)	250
Snickers	280	Iced-tea (20 oz Bottle)	200
Milky way	250	Snapple (20 oz Bottle)	240
Twix	280	Water	0
Starburst	240		
3 Musketeers	260	**PIZZA**	**CALORIES**
Skittles	250	Regular Pizza (Slice):	310 – 370
Reese's	230	Pizza Hut Pizza (Slice)	200
M & M'S Plain or Peanuts:	235 – 280	Little Caesars (Slice)	330
Kit Kat	220	Domino's Pizza 14" (Slice)	272
Hershey's	230	Papa John's Pizza 14" (Slice)	300
Nestle Crunch	220		
FRUITS & VEGETABLES	**CALORIES**	**McDONALD'S**	**CALORIES**
Apple	70	Burgers:	
Banana	105	• Hamburger	250
Grapefruit	80	• Cheeseburger	300
Grapes	75	• Double Cheeseburger	440
Orange	80	• Big Mac	540
Pear	80	• McChicken	360
Plum	40	• Quarter Pounder	410
Broccoli (1/2 cup)	25	French Fries:	
Carrot (1/2 cup)	35	• Small/Medium/Large	250/360/540
Cauliflower (1/2 cup)	15	Egg McMuffin	300
Celery (1 Piece)	2	Milk Shake (Small)	400
Corn (Ear)	95	Pancakes (2)	600
Cucumber	45	Deluxe Breakfast	1100
Lettuce (1 cup)	8		
Potato	75	**KFC**	**CALORIES**
Tomato	20	Chicken Pot Pie	770
		Cole Saw (1 serving)	190
		Crispy Stripes (3 Pieces)	400

SNACK FOODS	CALORIES	Chicken Breast (1 Piece)	440
Potato Chips (1oz)	150	Chicken Drumstick (1 Piece)	160
Pretzels (1oz)	110	Chicken Thigh (1 Piece)	370
Doritos (1 oz)	140	Honey BBQ Wings (6 Pieces)	540
Butter Popcorn (1oz)	160	Macaroni and Cheese	180
Cookies (2)	110-150	Mash Potatoes with Gray	130
Donuts (1)	210-260	Potato Wedges (Small)	240
Apple Pie (4 oz)	280	**SUBWAY**	**CALORIES**
Cake (3 oz)	305	Ham (6"/No Cheese)	290
Ice Cream (1/2 cup)	160	Roast Beef (6"/No Cheese)	290
IHOP	**CALORIES**	Turkey (6"/No Cheese)	280
Pancakes Short Stack (3)	330	Veggie Delite (6"/No Cheese)	240
Pancakes Full Stack (5)	550	**CHINESE FOOD**	**CALORIES**
Country Fried Steak/Eggs	1530	Egg roll (1)	200
Rooty Tooty Fresh and Fruity	855	Spring roll (1)	100
Omelet with (3) Pancakes	1200-1400	BBQ Spare Rib (4)	600
BBQ Bacon Cheeseburger w. Fries	1510	Fried Rice (1 cup)	320
Chicken Clubhouse Stacker w Fries	1710	French Fries	600
Patty Melt with Fries	1480	4 Chicken Wings and Fried Rice	1120
Ham & Egg Melt w. Onion Rings	1350	4 Chicken Wings and French Fries	1400

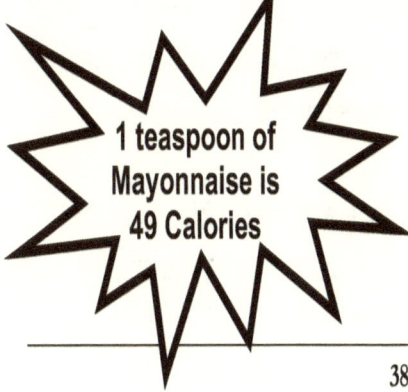

1 teaspoon of Mayonnaise is 49 Calories

HOW TO CUT YOUR CALORIES AND LOSE WEIGHT

You need to cut 3500 calories from your diet to lose 1 pound. So, if you cut out 500 calories a day from your daily eating in 7 days you will lose 1 pound. That's 1 pound a week, which is increased when you include exercise.

- If you eat 1 bag of potato chips a day for 7 days, that's 150 calories a day and 1050 calories a week. So, instead of eating 7 bags of potato chips a week eat 4 bags, which equal 600 calories and that cuts out **450** calories a week.

- If you eat 1 candy bar a day for 5 days, that's 280 calories a day and 1400 calories a week. So, instead of eating 5 candy bars a week eat 2 candy bars, which equals 560 calories and that cuts out **860** calories a week.

- If you eat a Big Mac, a large order of french fries and a soda once a week that's 1360 calories. Instead of having the above meal order a cheese burger, a small fries and a bottle of water, which equals 550 calories and that cuts out **810** calories a week.

- If you eat an order of 4 chicken wings and french fries from the Chinese restaurant that's 1400 calories. Instead of having the above meal order two spring rolls (200) and fried rice (320), which equals 520 calories and that cuts **880** calories a week.

- If you eat 2 slices of pizza a week and a soda that's 870 calories. Instead eat 1 slice of pizza and a water, which is 310 calories and that cuts **560** calories a week.

So, here is what we are looking at with minor cut backs in our daily diet:

450+860+810+880+560=3560, which is 1 pound of weight loss.

BEST WAY TO LOSE WEIGHT

- Cut calories and exercise
- Use smaller bowls, plates and cups when eating. This cuts the food portions.
- Buy smaller portions. You only eat big portions because you buy them. If you buy smaller portions you will satisfy your hunger or craving. Most of the time we eat not because we are hungry but because we see the food. Other times we mistake our body's craving for water, as a craving for something to eat.
- Drink water instead of soda or soft drinks.
- When you think you're hungry, have a glass of water, and many times you will no longer feel hungry.
- Eat more fruits, vegetables and nuts. You will grow to love them over time. Your taste buds will adjust to the healthier choices.

HOW MANY CALORIES DO YOU EAT A DAY?

Using the calories in food chart on pgs.37-38 and the internet, give an estimate of how many calories you consume a day. Write down the food and the amount of calories. Then add all of the calories and write down the total.

FOOD	CALORIES
TOTAL:	

Using the calories in food chart on pgs.37-38 and the internet, write down the amount of calories you would like to consume each day and the food you want to eat to help you reach your goal.

FOOD	CALORIES
TOTAL:	

5

EXERCISE IN THE INNER-CITY

****

CONSULT A PHYSICAN BEFORE CONDUCTING ANY EXERCISES, ESPECIALLY IF YOU HAVE A MEDICAL CONDITION.

EXERCISE IN THE INNER-CITY

Is there anywhere to exercise in the inner-city? Well, my mother lived in the projects in Brooklyn for 10 years and there were many exercise activities that could be done. The key is to be resourceful. Below is a list of free exercise activities you can do without spending money for a fancy gym membership:

- Climbing stairs – every project, and tenement dwelling has more than enough stair cases. You can make them your "StairMaster", and burn a lot of calories climbing the stairs. For safety precautions, this should be done in the daytime, and preferably with an exercise partner.
- Pull-ups on the Monkey Bars - if this activity is permitted, give it a try. If you are new to this exercise, it takes some getting use to.
- Jumping rope - this exercise is not just for little girls and teenagers. Jumping rope burns a lot of calories.
- Push-ups and Crunches.
- Walking or Jogging – you can start a walking or jogging club.

ESTIMATE CALORIES BURNED DURING EXERCISING

EXERCISE	MINUTES			
	15	30	45	60
Bike Riding	130 Cal.	260 Cal.	390 Cal.	520Cal.
Walking	75 Cal.	150 Cal.	275 Cal.	300 Cal.
Jogging	135 Cal.	270 Cal.	405 Cal.	540 Cal.
Skateboarding	95 Cal.	190 Cal.	285 Cal.	380 Cal.
Basketball	125 Cal.	250 Cal.	375 Cal.	500 Cal.
Baseball	50 Cal.	100 Cal.	150 Cal.	200 Cal.
Football	125 Cal.	250 Cal.	375 Cal.	500 Cal.
Swimming	125 Cal.	250 Cal.	375 Cal.	500 Cal.
Dancing	75 Cal.	150 Cal.	275 Cal.	300 Cal.
Tennis	125 Cal.	250 Cal.	375 Cal.	500 Cal.
Weights	70 Cal.	140 Cal.	210 Cal.	280 Cal.
Aerobics	125 Cal.	250 Cal.	375 Cal.	500 Cal.
Stair climbing	125 Cal.	250 Cal.	375 Cal.	500 Cal.

SAMPLE 7 DAY FOOD AND EXERCISE LOG

Breakfast	Exercise	Food	Exercise
Bowl of oatmeal	Bike 30 min	150	260
Wheat toast		120	
Orange Juice		90	
Banana		60	
Lunch			
Pizza			
Soda	Basketball	370	250
	30 minutes	250	
Dinner			
McDonald's			
Hamburger		250	
Small Fries		250	
Water		-0-	
Snacks			
Banana		105	
Orange		80	
Total Calories for Food and Exercise:		1725	510

SEE NEXT PAGE FOR EXPLANATION

If this was a real scenario of your routine for the day, how many calories did you consume? Let's break it down:

Your total calories consumed was: 1725

Your total calories burned was: 510

Now, deduct the calories burned from the calories consumed

That means: 1730 – 510 = 1215

Therefore, your calorie intake for the day is: **1215**

**Provided on pages 47-51 are 7 blank workout
logs to assist you with tracking your weekly
food consumption and exercise.**

BLANK WORKOUT LOG FOR DAY 1

Breakfast	Exercise	Food	Exercise
Lunch			
Dinner			
Snacks			
Total:			

CALORIES CONSUMED:_____

CALORIES BURNED:_____

CALORIES CONSUMED – CALORIES BURNED =:_____

TOTAL CALORIES FOR THE DAY:_____

BLANK WORKOUT LOG FOR DAY 2

Breakfast	Exercise	Food	Exercise
Lunch			
Dinner			
Snacks			
Total:			

CALORIES CONSUMED:_____

CALORIES BURNED:_____

CALORIES CONSUMED – CALORIES BURNED =:_____

TOTAL CALORIES FOR THE DAY:_____

BLANK WORKOUT LOG FOR DAY 3

Breakfast	Exercise	Food	Exercise
Lunch			
Dinner			
Snacks			
Total:			

CALORIES CONSUMED:_____

CALORIES BURNED:_____

CALORIES CONSUMED – CALORIES BURNED =:_____

TOTAL CALORIES FOR THE DAY:_____

BLANK WORKOUT LOG FOR DAY 4

Breakfast	Exercise	Food	Exercise
Lunch			
Dinner			
Snacks			
Total:			

CALORIES CONSUMED:_____

CALORIES BURNED:_____

CALORIES CONSUMED – CALORIES BURNED =:_____

TOTAL CALORIES FOR THE DAY:_____

BLANK WORKOUT LOG FOR DAY 5

Breakfast	Exercise	Food	Exercise
Lunch			
Dinner			
Snacks			
Total:			

CALORIES CONSUMED:_____

CALORIES BURNED:_____

CALORIES CONSUMED – CALORIES BURNED =:_____

TOTAL CALORIES FOR THE DAY:_____

BLANK WORKOUT LOG FOR DAY 6

Breakfast	Exercise	Food	Exercise
Lunch			
Dinner			
Snacks			
Total:			

CALORIES CONSUMED:_____

CALORIES BURNED:_____

CALORIES CONSUMED – CALORIES BURNED =:_____

TOTAL CALORIES FOR THE DAY:_____

BLANK WORKOUT LOG FOR DAY 7

Breakfast	Exercise	Food	Exercise
Lunch			
Dinner			
Snacks			
Total:			

CALORIES CONSUMED:_____

CALORIES BURNED:_____

CALORIES CONSUMED – CALORIES BURNED =:_____

TOTAL CALORIES FOR THE DAY:_____

TOTAL CALORIES FOR THE WEEK_____

EXERCISE

Get in shape with a low cost resistance band that you can purchase from a sports store and use the exercises shown on the following pages. 15 minutes, 1 set of 8-10 reps of each exercise and three days a week is all you need. Before conducting any of the following exercises do a 5 minute warm-up, which is included in your workout time. The warm-up should consist of running in place, jumping jacks and side bends. After you complete the exercises, cool down by stretching your muscles for approximately 2 minutes.

Resistance Band Exercises

Various resistance band exercises are included on the following pages, which includes exercises for:

- Arms (Bicep Curls and Tricep Kickbacks)
- Chest (Chest Press)
- Back (Bent Over Rows)
- Shoulders (Upright Rows)
- Legs (Squats)

RESISTANCE BAND EXERCISE – ARMS

BICEP CURLS

START

FINISH

Stand with the resistance band under your feet as you hold the handles with both hands. Slowly curl your arm by bending your elbow toward your shoulder. Slowly return to the starting position.

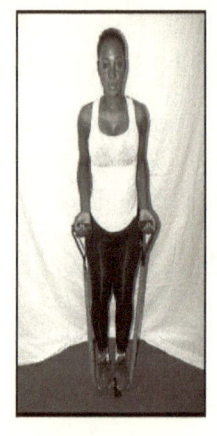
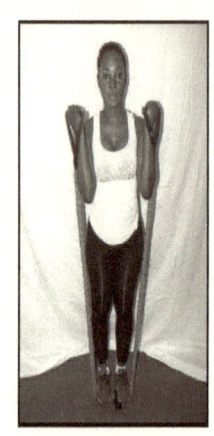

TRICEP KICKBACKS

START

FINISH

Stand with the resistance band under your feet as you hold the handles with both hands so that your elbows are close to your body. Slowly straighten your arms. Slowly return to the starting position.

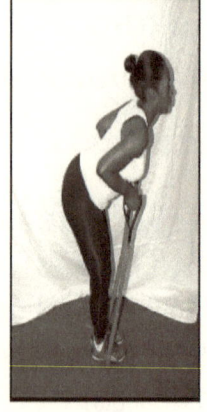
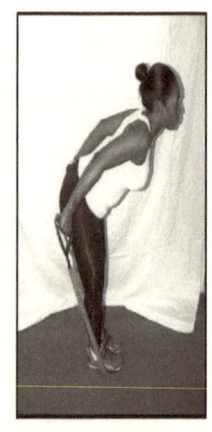

RESISTANCE BAND EXERCISE - CHEST

CHEST PRESS	START	FINISH	SIDE VIEW

Wrap the resistance band around your back. Grip both ends of the handles. Slowly press your arms forward. Slowly return to the starting position.

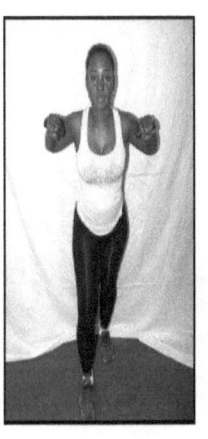
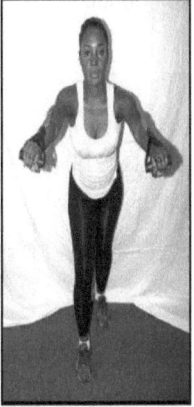
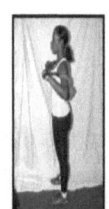
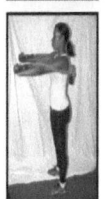

RESISTANCE BAND EXERCISE - BACK

BENT OVER ROW	START	FINISH

Stand with the resistance band under your feet as you hold the handles with both hands. Bend forward at the waist. Slowly pull the band up toward your chest. Slowly return to the starting position.

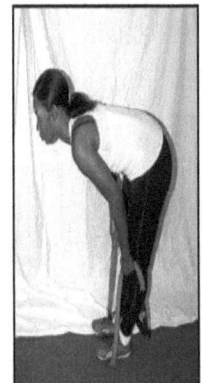
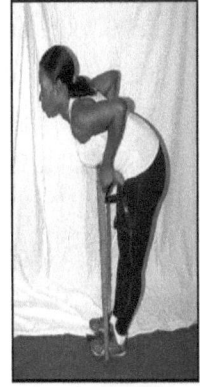

RESISTANCE BAND EXERCISE - SHOULDERS

UPRIGHT ROWS   START   FINISH

Stand with the resistance band under your feet as you hold the handles with both hands. Criss-cross the band in front of you. Pull your elbows up towards your chin. Slowly return to starting position.

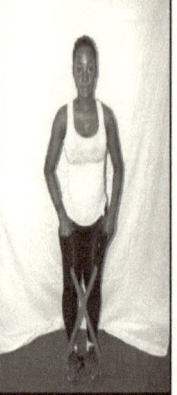
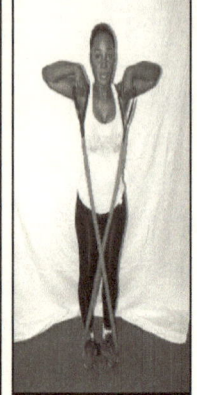
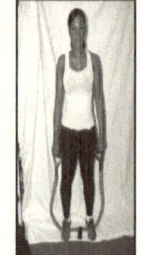
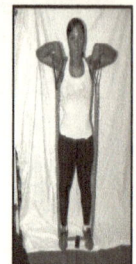

RESISTANCE BAND EXERCISE - LEGS

SQUATS   START   FINISH

Stand with the resistance band under your feet as you hold the handles with both hands at shoulder length. Slowly squat down. Slowly return to starting position.

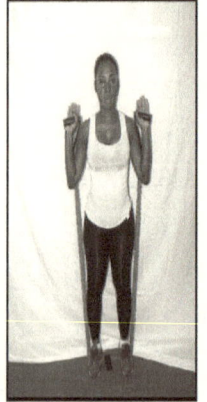
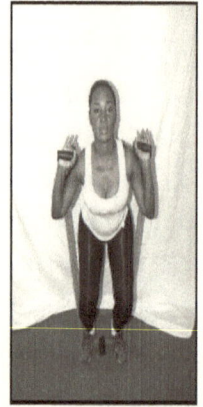

6

SALT, SUGAR & FRIED FOOD

SALT, SUGAR & FRIED FOOD

Salt consumption in inner-city communities are extremely high, so this is an issue that has to be addressed. High salt intake causes high blood pressure, headaches and numerous other ailments. In the inner-city, we have developed taste buds that crave spicy foods. If you do not believe me, go to a high-end restaurant and order something. When you receive the food you will immediately notice that it is bland. This is due to our high salt intake, which we have become addicted to. Besides adding salt to our food, we also use hot sauce to spice up our meal. Basically, hot sauce is salt.

High blood pressure is often called "the silent killer" since there are typically no symptoms. Undiagnosed, untreated high blood pressure, also known as hypertension ultimately leads to stroke, heart failure and other diseases.

THE SIDE EFFECTS OF SUGAR

Besides salt, sugar is one of the major hazards to our health. It is easy for us to exceed our daily sugar intake, which the AHA recommends 25 grams for women and 38 grams for men a day. For example, if you drink a soda (32 grams of sugar), eat a slice of cake (20 grams of sugar) you have went over the recommended sugar intake per day. The majority of restaurants that cater to urban areas put sugar in their foods because they know we like the sweet taste. Sugar has no positive benefits and causes the following ailments:

- Diabetes
- Obesity
- Depression
- Mood Swings

We have to be mindful that most of the food we eat and what we drink contain sugar as a base ingredient. When we cut back on our sugar intake, we improve our overall health. Replace your sugar cravings with low-sugar healthy fruits.

THE SIDE EFFECTS OF FRIED FOOD

Fried food, margarine and butter serve the same purpose and that is to clog up our arteries and cause strokes and heart attacks. Food deep fried in oil and coated with margarine and butter are high in fat and also promotes weight gain. Along with the above ailments, fried food increases LDL cholesterol, which is bad cholesterol, and raises blood pressure due to clogged arteries. Clogged arteries cause heart attacks. It is just that simple. Eating poorly on a consistent basis eventually results in major health issues that will negatively affect the quality of your life, and ultimately shorten your life span.

Fried food, margarine and butter may taste good but, once again, they are no good for you. Particularly, in the quantities that we have grown accustomed to. Margarine is loaded with chemicals and bleach. So, if you must have that butter flavor, use plant-based butter. It is all natural and in the health-food section of your grocery store.

7

THE NEW YOU

THE NEW YOU

By applying the information in this book to your life you can create a new you. The new you will make wiser choices when it comes to your health and well-being. You will eat the right foods and drink the right beverages that help promote a vibrant life. You can create a life free from chronic ailments like high blood pressure, diabetes and high cholesterol, which can be lowered by changing your eating and exercise habits.

By exercising and making small changes to what and how much you eat and drink, you will be able to lose weight and become healthier. You do not have to change your entire life all at once, but with gradual changes you can change your entire life forever.

Welcome to the

NEW YOU!

WHAT DID YOU LEARN FROM THIS BOOK?

_____

_____

_____

_____

_____

_____

WHAT CHANGES WILL YOU MAKE TO HELP IMPROVE YOUR HEALTH?

_____

_____

_____

_____

_____

_____

PROMISE LETTER TO MYSELF

I, _____on this ___day of _____ year_____,

promise to cut back on eating junk food, drinking soda and unhealthy

soft drinks. I will eat more fruits and vegetables and drink more water

from this day forward, so that I can live a long and vibrant life. I, also,

vow to exercise _____ times a week, so that I can improve my

health.

Signature

_____

OTHER BOOKS BY THE AUTHOR

All books available at www.helpchanges.org

- How to for Teens
- How to for Teens - Conflict Resolution
- Positive Luggage
- Secret Book of Quotes Part 1
- The Plan Inside Out
- Billy the Bully
- No More Cs
- Don't take Candy from Strangers
- Lost in the Mall
- Don't Play with Matches
- A Trip Around the House
- What Should I Eat?
- Change the Batteries